Make it a Great Journey

Amy A. Brothers

ISBN: 978-0-578-81928-0

GREENVILLE, NC

Book Project Management—RAINDROP CREATIVE | START WRITE PUBLISH
Cover Design—Brittany O. Annis/Rainah Davis
Illustrator: Brittany O. Annis
Start Write Editors: Gerald C. Simmons/Dr. Erin Almond
Start Editorial Assistant: Jennifer Eiland
Layout Designer: Pankaj Runthala

Dedication

I dedicate this book to each individual who has ever struggled with their weight. Don't give up. You can do it....let's make it a great journey!

TABLE OF CONTENTS

CHARTING YOUR PATH

Prologue

My Story

During most of my life, I have been blessed to have been surrounded by an abundance of family and friends. I come from humble beginnings with a big, loving country family; consisting of nine siblings and parents who had been married fifty-three strong years before Papa's passing. My father and brothers played a significant role in building my self-esteem and confidence. The men in my life loved me and always told me that I was beautiful and smart. Indeed, my family made me feel loved, safe and accepted. As a child, I had fat, round, chubby cheeks that would often get pinched by relatives at family gatherings. Family gatherings were special events and always included large helpings of Southern food, sweet tea or red punch, rich chocolate cakes, and lemon cakes. Because of the abundance of a warm, loving family and food to match, I have been known to be a happy, joyful person, full of spunk, spice, and life. I was a typical Southern gal: full-figured, bouncy, sweet as Dixie Crystal sugar, and the type who made "hey y'all" and a smile my standard greeting. I loved life and loved my plus-sized skin. I truly enjoyed the love of family, mostly when the gathering was around food.

The dinner table was a cornucopia-like event for my family. We would have "food aplenty," which meant no limits. All that was lacking was a printed sign above the table which read: "Eat as much as you want...there's plenty to go around!" My parents had a farm most of their lives: pigs, chickens, goats, horses, corn, sweet potatoes— you name it, we had it, and we had it "in plenty." We didn't run out of food because my father made sure there was an endless supply. My father, who grew up in the South in the 1930s, wanted his children to work hard, get a solid education, and never worry about essential things in life such as food, shelter, security, and being loved. My father was a stickler for keeping food in good supply and on our dinner table. He never wanted us to go hungry or worry about where our next meal would come from. Having been raised in the South, he himself had experienced nights of hunger and uncertainty. However, I never felt deprived of anything —especially food. My mother customarily cooked dinner every evening, and every Sunday morning, we would eat breakfast together as a family. Large thick slices of country bacon, pork sausage, enormous helpings of scrambled eggs with cheddar cheese, fried potato cakes, homemade Southern-style biscuits smothered in molasses, butter or grape jelly, and homemade pancakes with heavy Karo syrup. That meal's menu was a rich normalcy for me. When my parents sold the farm and slowly became more modernized, I began to look forward to Fridays when we would have pizza, which was a special treat. Soda, Kool-Aid, potato chips', cheese doodles, Little Debbie cakes, and ice cream became staple items inside our home, and I could eat them whenever I wanted —even for breakfast. No-one stopped me: my parents wanted me to be happy; therefore, we had "food aplenty."

Continuous availability of "food a plenty" took its toll on my outward appearance. Going to school as an over-weight child would have been a nightmare without my family and supportive childhood friends: Casey, Jillian, and Ashley. We didn't have external commonalities. We didn't see our differences but enjoyed each other's friendly, warm, outgoing personalities. No matter how solid the foundation and surroundings which one may have, children, however, can be cruel. For instance, I didn't know that anything was "wrong" with me until maybe the third or fourth grade - a point at which I began getting teased about my weight, which caused me to be much larger than an average-sized child my age. By the time I was in the fifth grade, I had weighed in at 175 pounds. Because of my weight, I physically developed early, and I had breasts by third grade (I got teased about those, as well). Because of my girth and height, I often had to "get in the back" while taking school pictures. Children poked fun and reminded me that I wasn't "normal," that I was "different," that I was — well, FAT. My being obese was not easy, and the teasing and words hurt and made me fearful. I would cringe whenever the teacher stepped out of the classroom because that's when the most substantial amount of the teasing began. I would hope that the bullies would pick someone else—anyone else but me, but fat jokes tended to be infamous crowd-pleasers and I happened to be an obvious target. Being teased and bullied would sometimes distract me from the classroom listening, so I made it a practice to read several chapters ahead of the class and complete my work in advance.

Nevertheless, fate was kind to an extent; I began to find joy in being proactive and ahead of everyone else. This advantage brought self-fulfillment and buttressed my damaged self-esteem. Moreover, I didn't let bullying stop me. I excelled in every area of study and became recognized for my advancement so overwhelmingly that it superseded my outward appearance. Also, I began to break the school norms: I tried out for the cheering squad during my fifth-grade year at Central Elementary. Trying out under the scrutiny of the eyes of the panel of judges was scary, but I had always wanted to be a cheerleader, and my family supported me. I tried out and made the squad! I was the first plus-sized cheerleader for the Central Elementary Wildcats. Subsequently, I was at every practice, in all the parades; and made friends wherever I went. I never knew how much of an impact I was making until other young overweight girls tried out the following year. As a result, I was selected to be a peer helper and began to help other students/peers with their self-esteem challenges: I had a chance to counsel them one-on-one or peer-to-peer.

By this time, I did not let my weight stop me from pursuing my dreams. Trying out for that cheering squad and making the team set off a line of fire that blazed throughout my adult life. I was courageous and limitless. I loved being *me*. I liked breaking barriers and challenging the norm. I enjoyed going to the beach and feeling free to wear bathing suits – unashamed. I began to enjoy theme parks with roller coasters and boat rides, festivals, and random road trips with friends —all of which included food. By the time I was in high school, I had weighed 250 pounds. Still, my life was surrounded by food and I loved to eat! I had a bubbly personality that attracted people. I had an enormous group of friends, went to prom with my high school sweetheart, and likewise, had boyfriends and heartbreaks like anyone else. (I was fat... not ugly!)

What is more, I was voted "best personality" during my senior year. I was accepted. And I enjoyed life. By the time I was in my freshman year of college, I had gained another 50 pounds, becoming 300+ pounds. I was 18-years-old and labeled morbidly obese. My weight and eating habits were out of control. In 2013 at age 31, I began having issues with varicose veins— my legs would fall asleep while I was sitting at my work desk. My legs would be swollen at the end of the day; they would bulge, and my calves would swell. The blood was not flowing correctly. My mother, who weighed approximately 400 pounds, had this same issue. However, she also had diabetes; her left leg had turned dark from lack of blood flow; she has high blood pressure, low heart rate, and is prescribed numerous medications. My blood pressure was always between 115/65, so there were so no "real issues" with my health. In 2014, I had a couple of scares. I began passing out randomly. My heart was required to be temporarily monitored. At this point, I weighed 325 pounds.

GUIDEPOST #1:

FUTURE SUCCESS OR FUTURE FAILURE

It is estimated that three million visitors hike a portion of the Appalachian Trail each year. Most enjoy day hikes and short backpacking trips, but each year, a small fraction of those hikers complete the entire Trail. Since 1936, more than 20,000 hike completions have been recorded by the Appalachian Trail Center.. That is only a tiny fraction of completions based on the number of hikers. The Appalachian Trail is 2,190 miles, and it takes five to seven months to complete the entire trail. It's no amateur hike!

It takes proper planning, preparation, and strategy. Before a hike, you must prepare by mapping out the appropriate route to take, how much food and supplies to pack for the journey, and check and re-check weather forecasts and prepare for obstacles that you may encounter along the way. To complete a hike on the Appalachian Trail, you must prepare to go the distance! Taking a 5-minute walk around the block is not equally comparable to hiking the Appalachian Trail. Both of these tasks require different amounts of time and effort. A smart approach to any project is thorough research, proper preparation and planning, and a solid strategy.

Likewise, I approached my planning for weight loss surgery in that same way. I will discuss more planning techniques throughout the next few chapters. I visualized the end result of my journey. The end for me with weight loss surgery was seeing a complete, happier, healthier version of myself. I imagined myself winning at the end of the journey. I defined winning as seeing my best self at a weight loss of 100 pounds, having established healthy eating and exercise habits, and a toned and defined body in which I would be satisfied. I understood that if I wanted to have and maintain this new version of myself, it would take hard work! I was determined to go the distance! How determined are you to go the distance with your weight loss journey? Are you willing to plan, prepare, and create a strategy to win and meet your goals? When considering weight loss surgery, it is crucial to understand the pros and cons of the decision and the many decisions you will make going forward. It is helpful to begin by doing a self-assessment and asking yourself the following questions:

- Should I have weight loss surgery?
- What do I need to do to start planning for weight loss surgery?
- Do I meet the physical requirements for weight loss surgery?
- Which weight loss surgery is the right one for me?
- Do I have the resilience and determination to keep going even if I run into a setback?

Taking time to do a self-assessment is vital to your success. All of the above questions will come to mind as you begin the bariatric process. Bariatrics describes the medical treatment of being seriously overweight—that is, obesity. Bariatric surgery is only employed when other methods of weight loss have been tried and failed. If you're like me, you have attempted every diet, meal plan, and fasting technique possible. Also, like me, you may have had in your possession multiple, unused gym memberships that continued to be drafted out of your bank account monthly. You may have signed up for "Sergeant-Slaughter-styled" boot camps or spent your vacation time at a "fat farm" (I did, and yes, they do exist!). You may also have binge-watched "My 600lb Life" —all out of desperation to get motivated to lose weight. Each of these examples mentioned illustrates crazy attempts to get us to snap ourselves out of whatever temptation holds us back from deciding to become our very best selves. If you have done any of the things mentioned above, then we have much in common. I hope that through my experiences and failures, you will be guided along your chosen path. My goal in penning this book is to help you build a strategy to win and have a successful bariatric weight loss journey. I hope you will embrace the fact that with every sacrifice made, there is a positive gain. You have the time. You have the ability. You can make an effort, and you will receive what you set out to achieve!

GUIDEPOST #2:

KNOW YOUR WHY

"Achievement happens when we pursue and attain what we want. Success comes when we are in clear pursuit of why we want it" - Simon Sinek

One of my favorite thought leaders is Simon Sinek. He wrote the *New York Times* bestseller "Start With Why." In the book, Simon discusses the influence of long-term success and what keeps us pursuing our goals. What is it that gives us the internal fortitude to continue on a path even when the course continues to get challenging or difficult? Simon references the importance of knowing and understanding your "why." *Why* is defined as "for what reason, cause, or purpose." Your *why* is the influencer and motivator for long-term success for your bariatric journey. The next step along the path is securing your *why*.

Based on research from the American Society for Metabolic and Bariatric surgery (ASMB), some of the top reasons individuals choose to have weight-loss surgery are morbid obesity, sickness, and/or disease. Each of these categories threatens a person's quality and length of life. Like many, I fell into the category of *obesity*. *Obesity* is a chronic disease that requires lifelong treatment and medical care. From self-consciousness to physical limitations, many people think that their size keeps them from being the person they truly are. A quote from one of my favorite proverbs is, "As a man thinketh, so is he." If an obese person believes that their physical appearance limits them from achieving what he/she hopes to obtain in their lifetime, then his/her belief in that thought will definitely be their determining limitation. People who are overweight are also at higher risk for developing severe health problems, such as heart disease, diabetes, high blood pressure, high cholesterol, stroke, arthritis, and gallbladder disease. *Obesity* is one of the underlying causes of most major medical conditions.

The Center for Disease Control defines obesity as a weight that is higher than what is considered a healthy weight for a given height. Body Mass Index, or BMI, is used as a screening tool to define healthy weight categories. If you have a body mass index of 30 or higher, you are considered obese. I was in that category for years, but I learned that I didn't have to stay in that state of being. As I began learning more about the effects of being obese, the information empowered me to learn about the tools available to combat my obesity. Obesity is a complex health issue resulting from various causes and individual factors such as behavior and genetics. Behaviors can include physical activity, inactivity, dietary patterns, medication use, and other exposures; additional contributing factors include food and physical activity environment, education and skills, food marketing, and promotion.

Obesity is also associated with the leading causes of death in the United States and worldwide. At age thirty, I was beginning to experience slight tell-tale signs of future health issues with the poor circulation of blood flow appearing in my legs through the visual display of varicose veins. My family had a history of diabetes and high blood pressure. Because of this knowledge of my family's health history, my ultimate goal was to get ahead of the health challenges plaguing my family and break the cycle of obesity and related diseases. In my research, I found that bariatric surgeries result in long-term weight-loss success. Most studies demonstrate that more than ninety percent of individuals previously affected by severe obesity successfully maintain fifty percent or more of their excess weight loss following bariatric surgery. More than eighty percent of those affected by super severe obesity can maintain more than fifty percent excess body weight loss. This information impacted my confidence in my decision and encouraged me to learn more. The *New England Journal of Medicine* conducted a study in 2007 which concluded that weight-loss surgery is an effective treatment for metabolic syndrome, which includes several conditions such as high blood pressure, high blood sugar; high cholesterol; and obesity. As an effective treatment for metabolic syndrome, weight loss surgery (also known as metabolic surgery) has been shown to lower blood sugar levels effectively and to reduce the risk for diabetes; lower blood pressure; and to reduce the risk for heart disease; cure sleep apnea and acid reflux, and to alleviate joint problems. I was glad to learn this information since diabetes was an area of future concern for me, based on family history.

Further studies proved to be exceptionally encouraging. Studies at the University of Duke revealed that people who undergo weight-loss procedures live 3.4 years longer than those who need but do not have bariatric surgery. And while there are risks and complications associated with all surgeries, weight-loss surgery is relatively safe. It results in positive outcomes because most procedures are performed through small incisions, which result in less pain, and faster recovery is usually experienced (Duke Medicine).

Learning more about obesity and the success rates of bariatric surgery helped me to secure my *why*. As you are defining your goals and confirming your why, there may be lingering thoughts that may cause you to vacillate regarding your decision to have surgery or not. It took me two years to decide to go through with having gastric bypass surgery! I never had major surgery before. This would be my first major medical venture, and I was afraid, and I was scared. Numerous questions bombarded my mind: Is weight-loss surgery safe? When I go under the anesthesia's effects, will I even wake up because of my size? I've tried every weight-loss solution there is. Is this option really going to work for me? To calm my fears and become more confident about my decision, I knew that I had to locate answers for the "unknown." I had to do my research.

GUIDEPOST #3:

DO YOUR RESEARCH

"Research is what I'm doing when I don't know what I'm doing"
- Wernher von Braun

The most common questions that I usually get from most people on the fence about their surgery decision are: "Where do I start?" or "Which weight-loss surgery should I get?" When I don't know what I'm doing, I actively research to find answers. The more I researched the bariatric process, the more answers I found, the more questions I had. More knowledge usually gives you more confidence to move forward. More information gives you the opportunity to make smart, solid choices. In my research regarding the options available and types of weight loss surgeries to choose from, I wanted to know which one would work best. I wanted to know which surgery would work best for my age, sex, ethnicity, weight, height, and medical history. I wanted to make sure that my choice matched my core habits. For example: if the weight-loss surgery of choice meant that I could eat only salads or vegetables, then that would not work for me at all. I already knew that I would fail before starting! I'm a meat-eater. Protein abstinence was and still is non-negotiable. Therefore, I looked for a surgery option that would still allow me to enjoy this food category in a healthy way. If you're like me, you've tried everything everyone else was doing and failed miserably! The diet more than likely wasn't the best-designed plan or course of action to take. Although the plan may have worked for your friend or co-worker, it may not be the best route to take for your preferences and goals. The right plan matters! I was on a journey to discover which weight-loss path would serve me best and work for me in the long-term. Remember that the decision for weight loss surgery is a journey!

Which Procedure Is Right for Me?

Many interested in bariatric surgery are unsure of which bariatric surgical procedure to get and have several questions. The first is usually, "What exactly is bariatric surgery?" This initial question is usually followed with, "Which procedure is right for me?" Bariatric procedures cause weight loss by restricting the amount of food the stomach can hold, causing malabsorption of nutrients, or by a combination of both gastric restriction and mal-absorption (ASMBS). I chose to have bariatric surgery after many failed attempts at a variety of diet programs. Gaining knowledge about each procedure was essential to me because I like to understand my options. I wanted to learn as much as I could about bariatric surgery to make the best possible choice. I began to read more about the pros and cons of each type of procedure that was available. Based on this book's timing, the following are the top three weight-loss (bariatric) procedures conducted in the United States: gastric banding, gastric sleeve, and gastric bypass. Let's look at each one individually.

Adjustable Gastric Banding

What it is: *Gastric banding* is a type of restrictive weight loss surgery.

How it works: The surgeon uses an inflatable band to squeeze the stomach into two sections: a smaller upper pouch and a larger lower section. The two sections are still connected by a tiny channel which slows down the emptying of the upper pouch. Most people can eat only a 1/2 to 1 cup of food before feeling too full or sick. The food also needs to be soft or well-chewed (Mayo Clinic).

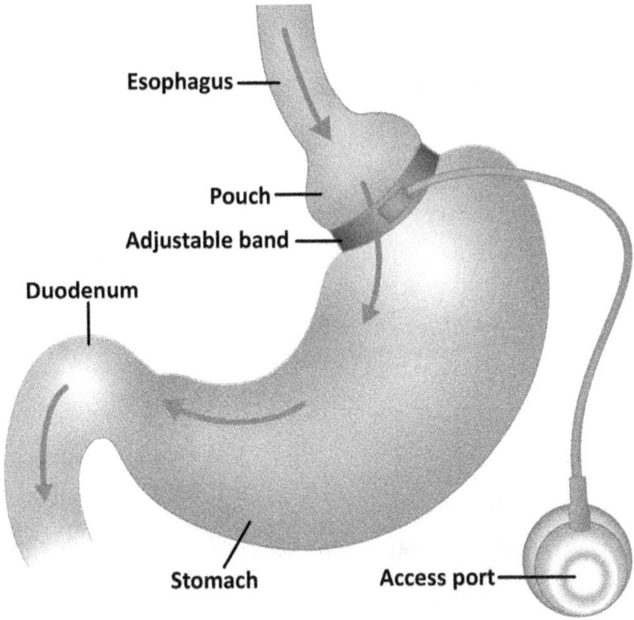

FIGURE 1

Pros: This operation is simpler to perform and safer than gastric bypass and other procedures. You get a smaller scar, recovery is usually faster, and you can have surgery to remove the band.

You can also get the band adjusted in a doctor's office. To tighten the band and further restrict your stomach size, the doctor injects more saline solution into the band. To loosen it, the doctor uses a needle to remove liquid from the band.

Cons: People who get gastric banding often have less dramatic weight loss than those who get other related surgeries. People who choose the gastric band option may also be more likely to regain some weight over the years.

Risks: One of the most common side-effects of gastric banding is vomiting after overeating too quickly. Complications with the band can happen. It might slip out of place, become too loose, or leak. Some people need more surgeries. As with any operation, infection is a risk. Although unlikely, some complications can be life-threatening (Mayo Clinic).

Sleeve Gastrectomy

What is it? Sleeve Gastrectomy is another form of restrictive weight-loss surgery. During the operation, the surgeon removes about seventy-five percent of the stomach. What remains of the stomach is a narrow tube or sleeve, which connects to the intestines. Sometimes, a sleeve gastrectomy is the first step in a series of weight-loss surgeries. For some people, it's the only surgery they need (Mayo Clinic).

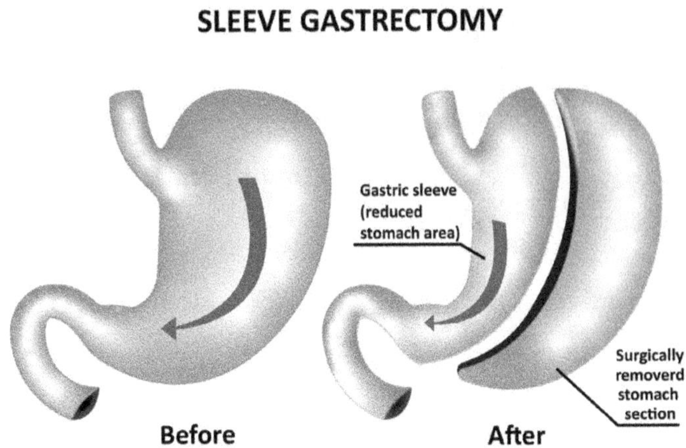

FIGURE 2

Pros: For people who are very obese or sick, other weight-loss surgeries may be too risky. A sleeve gastrectomy is a more straightforward operation that gives a lower-risk way to lose weight. If needed, once they've lost weight and their health has improved - usually, after 12 to 18 months, they can have a second surgery such as gastric bypass. Because the intestines aren't affected, a sleeve gastrectomy doesn't affect how your body absorbs food, so you're not as likely to fall short on nutrients (Mayo Clinic).

Cons: Unlike gastric banding, a sleeve gastrectomy is irreversible. Since it's relatively new, the long-term benefits and risks are still being evaluated.

Risks: Typical risks include infection, leaking of the sleeve, and blood clots.

Gastric Bypass Surgery (Roux-en-Y Gastric Bypass)

What is it? Gastric bypass combines both restrictive and malabsorptive approaches.

During the operation, the surgeon divides the stomach into two parts, sealing off the upper section from the lower. The surgeon then connects the upper stomach directly to the lower section of the small intestine. The surgeon is essentially creating a shortcut for the food, bypassing part of the stomach and the small intestine (See image). Skipping these parts of the digestive tract means that the patient's body absorbs fewer calories (Mayo Clinic).

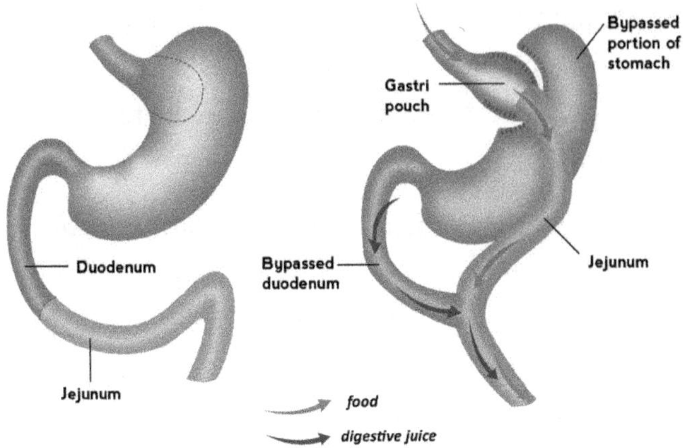

Figure 3

Pros: Weight loss tends to be swift and dramatic. About fifty percent of weight loss happens in the first six months. It may continue for up to two years after the operation. Because of the rapid weight loss, conditions affected by obesity — such as diabetes, high blood pressure; high cholesterol; arthritis; sleep apnea; and heartburn — often get better quickly. Gastric bypass also has good long-term results. Studies have found that many people keep most of the weight off for ten years or longer (Mayo Clinic).

Cons: You won't absorb food the way you used to, and absorbing food differently puts you at risk of not getting enough nutrients. The loss of calcium and iron could lead to osteoporosis and anemia. You will have to be very careful with your diet and take supplements for the rest of your life.

Another risk of gastric bypass is *dumping syndrome*, a condition in which food dumps from the stomach into the intestines too quickly before the food has been adequately digested. About eighty-five percent of people who undergo a gastric bypass have some dumping. Symptoms include nausea, bloating, pain, sweating, weakness, and diarrhea. *Dumping* is often triggered by eating sugary or high-carbohydrate foods. Adjusting your diet can often help.

Unlike adjustable gastric banding, gastric bypass is generally considered irreversible. However, it has been reversed in rare cases.

Risks: Because gastric bypass is more complicated, it is riskier. Infection and blood clots are risks, as they are with most surgeries. Gastric bypass also makes hernias more likely, which may create a need for further surgery to fix. Also, you may get gallstones because of rapid weight loss (Mayo Clinic).

So which weight loss surgery should you get?

The ideal weight-loss surgery depends on your health and body type. For instance, if you are very obese or have had abdominal surgery before, more straightforward surgeries might not be possible. Talk with your doctor about the pros and cons of each procedure. Go to a medical center that specializes in weight-loss surgery. Studies show that complications are less likely when weight-loss surgery is done by experts. No matter where you are, always ensure that your surgeon has had plenty of experience performing the procedure you need.

GUIDEPOST #4:

CONSULT OTHERS

Without counsel, plans fail, but with many advisers, they succeed. -Proverbs 15:22, ESV Bible

Whenever I'm in the process of "grinding" or thinking through an approach to something new, I seek out the experts. An expert can be a doctor, nurse, medical office staff, or persons who have had first-hand experience with weight-loss surgery. I have found that there is great wisdom in getting advice from others who are qualified!.

Gaining information saves a great deal of time, and it takes the worry out of the unknown. There is no way I could have gotten the information and support that I needed to make smart and informed decisions without the advice of professionals and those who have had experience with bariatric surgery.

Seek Professional Guidance

The next step on my journey was to speak to doctors' offices and obtain professional counsel. I wanted to get insight before hopping on YouTube and scaring myself to death by watching "weight loss surgery gone wrong" videos. I reached out to two offices in my local area highly rated on multiple websites and referrals from credible others. I signed up to attend their free group consultation classes. I gathered information from both offices and compared each of their doctors, along with their professional experience, insurance coverage offerings, process differences (not all offices are the same), and how well each office would follow up and follow through with me during the pre/post-Bariatric process. The items mentioned were vital to me as a patient. I asked questions surrounding those key components. Once each office answered my questions, and I attended their free consultation classes, I was ready to decide which practice would gain my business and me as a patient. Southern Surgical & Associates, located in Eastern North Carolina, stood out above the rest, and I selected this office as my health care provider for bariatric surgery. I chose Southern Surgical because of the experience the doctors in the office had with gastric bypass and sleeve options (which I wanted based on my research). The bypass and sleeve yielded the highest weight loss outcomes, with gastric bypass leading in weight loss results. As I began to go deeper into my journey and learned more about weight loss surgery, my mind began to shift and prepare for the journey and the life change ahead. I knew I had to get more information, so I decided to seek out those who had surgery with great success and those with failed results.

Reach Out to Others Who Have Had a Successful Experience

My next proactive step on my weight-loss journey was reaching out to others who had undergone the gastric bypass or gastric sleeve performed and learned about each of their experiences. But, "Where do you find them?" I found people in the small group consultation classes that I attended and inside my local church. I spoke to various age ranges, genders, and situation types: a married male in his thirties with four children; a fifty-year-old single mom, a forty-year-old single nurse (no children), a thirty-five-year-old married expectant mother (five children); the persons that I spoke with had great results and had kept the weight off. I learned from each of their stories the common denominators or areas of consistency. Each recounted their success and maintained weight loss by sticking with the bariatric diet plan issued by their doctors' office/dietician, taking bariatric vitamins religiously, and maintaining an exercise regimen. These persons were also very positive and practiced great self-talk, even if they had difficult days. I learned that discipline and consistency are required to stay on track. I understood that positive self-talk was something that I needed to continue to practice to make my weight loss plan a successful journey.

Have a Conversation With Those Who Have Had An Unsuccessful Experience

On my journey, I also met with those who had undergone weight-loss surgery and had gained their weight back.

Most would call substantial weight gain a failed surgery. I asked each person to find out some of the things that they felt that challenged them the most, and the typical answers were: stopped taking vitamins, didn't work out or feel the need to since the weight came off by itself; and several ate what they wanted whenever they wanted, even shortly after surgery. One of the scariest conversations around weight-loss surgery was speaking to a young lady in her late thirties who had the gastric sleeve performed. Let's call her Lucy. Lucy lost approximately seventy pounds after surgery. She loved to eat and cook fried Southern food and indulge in all of the richest desserts and southern delicacies. After almost three years post-surgery, Lucy had gained half her weight back. She shared with me that she would eat the fried foods and sweets, and then she would take herself to the bathroom and vomit it all back up.

Lucy began to chart her path on a bulimic-style behavior. Bulimia nervousa is an eating disorder in which a large quantity of food is consumed in a short period, often followed by feelings of guilt or shame. People with bulimia take steps to avoid weight gain and calorie intake by purging or vomiting. I found that Lucy's behavior was not only a weight challenge but a mental health issue as well.

After attending bariatric support group sessions myself, I heard stories just like Lucy's and understood that this behavior was not uncommon. I learned from Lucy that I needed to redefine how I thought about food and the importance of behavior modification. I began to plan my strategy to gradually remove fried foods and sweets before having surgery while on my journey to a healthier lifestyle. Another scenario was that of one of the males that I spoke with, named Bo, who had the gastric sleeve performed at the age of forty-three. Bo reminded me of a stocky football player with the grunt and grit in his personality to match. He was initially concerned about portion sizes and could not fathom moving from a large steak and potatoes helpings to a scaled-down petite plate of three ounces of salmon and light vegetables. Having a more petite plate didn't seem right to this alpha male who was accustomed to his steak and potatoes lifestyle. The small portion sizes were feminine to him and distinctively an odd behavior for an alpha male. This personally affected Bo's ego. He shared that he was often dizzy and experienced headaches due to eating so little. However, after digging a little deeper, Bo wasn't consistent with taking his vitamins, water consumption for hydration, and did not attend support groups. Bo initially fell back into his eating behaviors only eight months after his bariatric surgery.

Another story includes a married couple. A gentleman and his wife underwent gastric bypass at the same time. They were nearing fifty years of age and absolutely loved food. I had lunch with the couple before and after their surgeries. Pre-surgery, they were very obese. The husband weighed between 400-450 pounds, and the wife weighed between 250-300 pounds. Both had demanding lifestyles that required long hours and fluctuating schedules. When sitting at our lunch table and reviewing the menu, with the anticipation of food, the couple would get so excited that they would begin humming and singing at the lunch table. When the large portions of food would arrive, the couple would talk about each dish with such desire and affection that, had I not known it was food, I honestly would have thought it was the other's lover! Their passion for food was extreme. When they shared with me that they were going to have weight-loss surgery, I raised concerns regarding preparation for surgery, shared what I had learned, and questioned if they would shift their eating habits and diet before their surgery date. The couple did not see the need to adjust their behavior. Instead of changing their eating habits, the couple's approach pre-surgery was to gorge and eat all the unhealthy foods they loved. Because they knew that they might very well be removing several of the foods from their diet, the couple chose to eat all that they loved and as much as they possibly could leading up to their surgery. The couple treated their decision to have surgery as though they were having a long-term celebratory "goodbye" to their loved foods. I questioned this approach. For me, gorging on unhealthy foods would just make me want those foods that I couldn't have even more. However, everyone's path is their own.

Furthermore, once someone has his/her mindset or has decided, it is ultimately up to the individual how he/she may chart the path forward. I connected with the couple several months after their surgery. They had lost weight, and they both looked great! The couple did well for the first few months after weight loss, post-surgery; however, making good food choices was a severe challenge. Portion control was also still a significant struggle for the couple. Unfortunately, marital issues began to arise, and other life challenges came into play. The couple still maintained a demanding schedule but did not plan for or change their food choices. The couple fell back into poor food habits:

indulging in large portions, eating foods high in fat and carbohydrates. The couple also did not have an exercise routine before surgery and had no plans to work out post-surgery. They both began to regain their weight.

You may be asking yourself, "How could one still gain weight after undergoing bariatric surgery?" "Having bariatric surgery is a guaranteed weight loss win, right?" With anything worth having and keeping, there is more work, and there are more steps required to move forward and maintain progress. After having surgery, you still have an outstanding possibility to regain the weight. My doctor's office relayed that if you can maintain your weight beyond two years post-surgery, then you more than likely will not regain the weight lost. Individuals who have had weight loss surgery and gain their weight back often push past their triggers. *Triggers* are defined as the internal responses, both mentally and physically, limiting food intake and curve behavior. Triggers are behavior barriers gained from bariatric surgery that help support your decision not to overeat or have foods that could cause weight gain. These internal triggers are set in place to protect recovering bariatric patients from poor behaviors. For example, if a person who has undergone surgery ate at their food intake limit (which is approximately five to six ounces), their body would feel the physical reaction of being full. The physical reaction of being full would send a message to the brain, and the normal physical response would be to stop eating. Likewise, if a person who had surgery would eat something excessively filled with sugar and carbohydrates, their body would react with the feeling of nausea, dumping, or vomiting. The physical reaction would be the body, ultimately rejecting the food.

However, with gastric bypass, a person can mentally push past those triggers, even if their body responds with an adverse reaction or trigger. An example would be our friend Lucy who was mentioned earlier. Lucy would continue to eat unhealthy foods and retreat to the bathroom and vomit her food. Lucy continued to push past the triggered response and continued to eat those rich southern foods. Eventually, Lucy's body began to be conditioned to receiving the foods, and over time, she no longer vomited. Instead, her body adjusted to the fried foods and rich desserts. The body eventually will stop responding, turning off the triggers, and the person would then return to his/her poor eating habits and lifestyle.

I learned from other's experiences that along with surgery, a person's mental focus is essential. You must choose good and healthy habits. I also realized that I needed to change my language about food, not just how I thought about it. What is more, I couldn't talk about eating food as if it were an exciting event. I had to redefine food as fuel for my body to function correctly. I also attached greater importance for redefining my approach to dietary restrictions and changes. I had to become satisfied with not having the cookies, peach cobblers or chocolate cake, etc. If I did not take my lifestyle after surgery seriously, I could risk stretching out my new pouch (stomach). Stretching out your new pouch meant that you could eat more food, which is reversing the process for which it was intended. Making smart food choices and limiting portion size can prevent the extending of your pouch. Ultimately, weight-loss surgery didn't fail the groups or individuals mentioned. The choices we make, either good or bad, will cause our most significant success or future failure. As my mother would say, "It takes a 'made up mind' to complete a plan and stick to it." I valued the counsel of each of the individuals and groups mentioned because their insight helped me to make better choices on my journey to better health. I hope that these life lessons also help you with your future decisions!

GUIDEPOST #5:

MAKING THE DECISION

"The power to turn the bad into good, the good into great, and the great into amazing is in your hands."- Jeanette Jenkins, Hollywood Trainer/Health Coach

I've spoken to many men and women who have felt powerless when it comes to losing large quantities of weight. I understand and can relate to that feeling. I recall having that type of defeated mindset. I had even grown into accepting that maybe I was supposed to be overweight and to simply live with it since I had already done so for so long. I had tried every diet and starvation tactic known to mankind. My downfall was my level of discipline and consistency. If the plan or process didn't work fast enough, I was doubting and quitting. One of the key turning points for me was that I began to gain confidence through my research. I asked as many questions as possible to understand precisely what I was getting myself into, and I owned the fact I was going on a lifelong journey. If you're like me, you struggled hard with making the final decision to have surgery. The power is definitely in your hands, and you have control over your future. You can turn your current situation from good into great, and from great to extraordinary. With your decision, you must have settled these three things:

1. Weight loss surgery is not a quick fix.
2. You are not taking the "easy way out" by having weight-loss surgery.
3. You are not a failure, and you're not weak by choosing to have surgery.

Not A Quick Fix

Al Roker, weatherman for NBC's Today Show stated, "There's no quick fix (for weight loss). At the end of the day you still have to do the work to maintain your weight. It can't be a diet. You have to change your life." Weight-loss surgery is not a quick fix, but an invaluable tool if you're expecting long-term weight-loss results. A quick fix is something that's done generally to fix a short-term problem. A quick fix is much like getting a temporary plug for your vehicle tire when it goes flat. You know that the plug is there to hold your tire with air temporarily until you can get your vehicle into an auto shop to have your tire replaced. The new tire is suited for better long-term results. The same principle holds with weight-loss surgery, and the goal is to maintain this new lifestyle long-term.

Additionally, weight loss through bariatric means is a process and takes much discipline and consistency for your long-term health and best physical outcome. The personal responsibility of weight loss surgery takes disciplined eating, consistent workouts, and an overall healthy lifestyle to achieve full results. I must forewarn you if you are not prepared to commit to a new and healthy way of eating and living, you may lose the weight, but, unfortunately, you will also gain it back, along with several extra pounds.

Not Taking the Easy Way Out

You are not taking the easy way out by deciding to have weight-loss surgery. Surprisingly, many people struggle with weakness by accepting the help and benefits that bariatric weight loss has to offer. An example of weakness would be continuing to give in to the temptation of overeating. Making poor choices in what is being consumed can negatively affect your health. Acknowledging that you need help in an area of weakness and personal struggles take strength and courage. If your goal is to live a better quality of life, you must make decisions that align with your goals. You are not a failure for deciding to have surgery. In fact, you are learning from your past diets and putting the necessary boundaries and processes in place for a healthier, balanced future. Bear in mind that weight-loss surgery is a tool to be used for your benefit. In the earlier guidepost, I mentioned the importance of defining success for yourself. I shared that my definition of success included losing 140 pounds and being toned and satisfied with my body. I understood that it would take physical and mental work to maintain weight loss and to achieve satisfaction. Waking up at 4:30 AM for workouts, meal prepping on the weekends for the upcoming week, carrying lunch to work each day, and saying no to co-workers who bring in those desserts and homemade treats, are all a part of the "work" it takes to restructure your life and to put boundaries and processes into place. These are not always easy choices. It takes intentional decision making, discipline, and consistency to keep the result of your goals in focus.

You're Not A Failure

In 2015, I decided to have gastric bypass surgery. Before doing the research, I had to deal with my initial thoughts of surgery. My ego said that I could lose the weight on my own. At first, I took the initial idea of surgery off the table. But the grim, overshadowing vision of my future haunted me. I didn't want to be on a talk show in a purple moo-moo, crying hysterically, with a half-eaten Snickers bar in one hand and a carton of Ben & Jerry's ice cream in the other, dramatically wailing loudly, "I just can't stop eating!" This depiction of my out of control self is extreme, but hopefully, you get the picture!

I revisited the thought of surgery after I had a final wake-up call by my fainting - a condition that left me in the hospital in 2014. I was attending a formal event for my organization when I began to feel extremely warm mid-event. I began to sweat profusely, and my breathing started to get irregular. I needed to get some fresh air, so I stood up to take my exit. I got to the door to enter the main lobby, and I went face forward into the carpet. BOOM! I woke up moments later with cold compresses on my neck and wrist. An ambulance had been called. The EMT shared that my blood pressure was severely low, and it caused me to faint. He could not pinpoint my issue. I went to the hospital, and I was severely dehydrated, and my heart rate was low. The doctor had an IV installed to give me fluids. My main concern was my future health, and I agreed to begin researching and understanding the pros and cons of weight-loss surgery. No matter how many failed attempts that I had in the past with weight loss, my past was not going to predict my future. I decided to change the narrative. Changing the narrative started with a decision. Choosing to have weight-loss surgery gave me a sense of empowerment. I took control of my life and every overwhelming and self-defeating thought that was subconsciously running my life. I now had the power to change the trajectory of my story. Weight-loss surgery, for me, would be the tool used to help pioneer a new path for my family, rewrite its history, and open the door to more opportunities than I could have ever imagined, such as the ability to run a 5K, compete in sports, but most importantly, for me to be confident and satisfied with myself as an individual. Another reason that I chose the option of gastric bypass is that at the time, this procedure yielded the highest weight-loss results. Secondary weight-loss procedures were less common, and gastric bypass fitted most closely with my core eating behaviors. As mentioned previously, one of my core eating behaviors needed to include high protein in my diet. Because of my need for meat, I could adhere to the diet requirements and restrictions. Having gastric bypass required me to have 60 grams of protein per day with a strict limit of carbohydrates and sugar intake. Throughout this book, I will focus my attention on gastric bypass and my experience with it; however, many of the strategies and tools mentioned will help most who pursue bariatric surgery. My next steps were to select my support team.

GUIDEPOST #6:

YOUR SUPPORT TEAM

"Alone we can do so little; together we can do so much." – Helen Keller

If you have ever seen anyone achieve anything significant long-term, he/she did it with a team. Successful teams work together to achieve a common purpose or goal. Moreover, a good team will celebrate wins together and hold each other accountable for their actions. It is vital to surround yourself with people who are positive, encouraging, and available to you as you take on your new journey. Your support team will also continuously encourage you to go after your goals. You may want to slack off, and you will, but it is good to have strong supporters who care enough about you to tell you the truth and help you to get back on track. What does having a good support team look like?

For the most part, I kept my surgery quiet. Being a single female, I shared my decision with only a small group of individuals. I shared my decision in phases and with good timing. For those who were closest to me (my core), I shared my decision immediately. I then announced it to my co-workers and volunteer team a month before my leave so that they wouldn't be shocked when I returned and wonder, "Who is this person?" (weight loss occurs fast!). I didn't, however, share it with all of my immediate family members. Although I have a very supportive family, they are very traditional. My family would have echoed my initial concerns to me more often than I would have liked and possibly would have tried to get me to change my mind. They would have been a positive group of influencers against my having surgery, using such words like: "You look fine just like you are." "You really don't need to do this." Although they would have meant well and truly cared about my wellbeing, their opinions would have gone against my values and what I needed to do for myself at the time. I decided to keep any naysayers out of this decision. Selecting the right people to come alongside you on your journey plays such a significant role in the future of your success. These select persons must agree with your surgery choice, speak positively about your surgery, and be cheerleaders in your corner. Having a home supporter, medical specialist, and a food accountability partner are all key to the beginning stages of creating your team. My support team evolved over time as my needs changed.

The A-Team

Thankfully, my support team seemed to already be in place before I started planning. You may or may not have relationships in place that can surround you with support. I will share how I went about the selection process and what key roles each person took in my success. I started by writing down a list of prospective team members and slightly mentioned in conversation that I was considering weight-loss surgery. I asked each of them what they thought about weight-loss surgery. Each of them gave very positive responses, and I knew that I wanted them to be near when the time came for me to have gastric bypass.

My sister Nancy has supported me in everything that I have ever set my mind to do as an adult. She has graciously been in my corner and often would say, "If Amy said it, she's going to do it." At the time of my surgery, Nancy was living with me and committed to helping me at home post-operation. She was the MVP (most valuable player) of my support team. Nancy came along with me during support group sessions, and I introduced her to my doctors, along with making Nancy my emergency contact. She also had access to my files and was my medical power of attorney should anything have happened during my surgery that called for an interjection or answer. Then there was the nurse, Kathy, a good friend of mine and a registered nurse (RN) for over twenty years. She had gone through the process of bariatric surgery three years before my own and looked amazing! Kathy had spent a good bit of her time educating me on how to prepare for surgery. She gave me general expectations and how to navigate through difficult times. Kathy was wise and would tell me just enough to keep me focused and just enough not to scare me to death or have me running for the hills! She taught me how to listen to my body and adapt to the new changes that I would encounter. In brief, she was always available to answer any questions that I had. Kathy was and still is a great cheerleader in my corner. Then there was Holly. Holly was my third supporter, and I gave her permission to be my accountability partner. It's a good idea to give someone permission to call you out when you are making unwise choices in the early stages. "It sounds crazy now, but you'll thank me later!" seemed to be the attitudes of my guardian angels. You must grant someone permission to tell you "NO." Some may call this type of supporter "the voice of reason. I nicknamed her, "Hold 'Em, Holly."

After I had undergone surgery and had graduated to a regulated diet, Holly and I would be sitting at a table inside a restaurant and about to dig into an amazing meal that was overly portioned and questionable for a bariatric patient. "Hold 'Em Holly" would look at my plate, pointing her fork at me, and say, "Amy, are you *really* going to eat *all* of that?" Many times, as you're again learning how to eat and how to portion out your meals, you will make your plate as large as you had done before surgery purely out of habit. Habits are defined as an acquired behavior pattern regularly followed until it has become almost involuntary

(Webster). You will learn to break the habits of unhealthy eating as you continue your journey. In Charles Duhigg's book *The Power of Habits*, you break a habit by replacing the old harmful habit with a new, healthy, and positive one. One small thing that I adjusted was replacing my larger dinner plate with a smaller salad plate for all of my meals. I no longer own any large-sized plates since they no longer fit or serve my new lifestyle. The slight behavior change mentally kept me focused.

Holly would continue, with an eyebrow raised: "You already know what will happen if you eat all that—especially if you eat it way too fast." Holly had experienced seeing me "dump" several times after surgery. Believe me; it was more horrific for her to watch than it is for me to share. Dumping caused me to break out in a sweat, shaking/jitters, and the worst part was the vomiting. If the food's consistency or texture did not agree with me, or if I would eat too fast or too much, I would dump. If the food contains too much sugar, then the results are likely to be a fit of dumping. Sometimes, I didn't know when I was eating something that included large portions of sugar, such as condiments like ketchup, mayonnaise, barbecue sauces, etc. As a result, I would end up racing to the bathroom, often several times, in record speed so that it all could come up in the nearest toilet. Eventually, I began preparing more meals at home because I knew what ingredients and how much ingredients each meal contained.

Throughout the many similar ordeals, Holly remained a constant companion. I really appreciated this type of supporter! However, a "Hold 'Em Holly" was well needed as her voice began to stick with me when I was out on my own and having to make hard decisions about eating the right foods or not. You have to appreciate a friend like this who would firmly remind you of your goals and always stand as a strong encourager who will let you know that you still need to take the necessary steps to set required boundaries.

Intermediate Supporters

I also used this opportunity to build relationships that may have been in a crunch or strain. I found the best way to build a relationship is to go through something together. It could be something simple: reading a book together or participating in a new activity or sport. I included my sister Vanessa and her daughters. You may want to have your children or other family members who want to see you win! For me, it was my sixteen-year-old nieces who loved the fact that I was keeping a secret from my other brothers and sisters! —My nieces enjoyed the idea of having "inside information"! I would receive random text messages that would read: "You've got this!" "You're doing great!" "You inspire me." "I'm so happy for you! #TeamAmy!" What an incredible group of supporters this group ended up being as my body began to change!

Faith

My faith played a significant part in my success. Daily prayer, affirmations, and meditation kept me on the right path forward; since prayer is at the beginning of every life turn that I have made, I don't make decisions without aligning my heart and mind with God. Some may think, "Well, what does God or faith have to do with this?" Some of the individuals whom I have now coached and offered guidance shared with me that they were praying about losing weight and felt that if they had had surgery, then making this decision meant that they didn't have faith in God. I can say that prior to understanding, I could see how that way of thinking could be a challenge for anyone. The good news is that God has plans to prosper us, and His desire is for us to live in good health so that our soul prospers. God certainly is more than willing to help us along our path. If weight loss surgery is something you're using as a tool to live a better quality of life, then I think He is a gracious God Who cares about the things that we care about and is with us all of the way!

Medical Team

I had the best support team at Southern Surgical and Associates. Your doctor's office will play a major role in this part of the weight-loss process. If you have a supportive office to work with, they will help navigate you through each stage of the post-weight-loss process. A good doctor's office will answer your questions, share information on the next steps, and provide you with a plan to succeed throughout your process. Southern Surgical provided a team of doctors who specialized in bariatrics and had performed multiple surgeries. Therefore, the team was well-versed in old and new procedures and helped me find the most effective one. I was able to have conversations with the medical team, and they walked me through the insurance process, shared with me expectations, and provided a monthly support group session with experts who came in to share as well as being able to have conversations with veteran weight-loss surgery patients that attended the support group sessions. I encourage you to find a good support group. Although I respect Facebook, some of the information in the group chats are questionable. Please consult a professional team or someone who has gone through the surgery process while utilizing the help and services of a certified medical team.

Financial Investment

Counting the cost and understanding what it will take out of pocket will help with your resolve. *Resolve* is sticking with your weight-loss goals. Most people want to know the actual surgery's financial cost, but allow me to challenge you to think more about the long-term cost of having weight-loss surgery. Some items will be lifelong purchases: protein drinks, multi-vitamins, calcium, iron, D-3 are just a few of the core items needed for your health. Based on the types of vitamins you use, you will spend approximately $30-40 per month on vitamins. Depending on the type(s) of protein shakes, they may cost approximately $20 for a box of twelve. I'm sharing this information just to give you an idea of the long-term cost versus the immediate.

Having weight-loss surgery can be rather costly financially if you do not have insurance coverage. The average weight-loss surgery in the United States in 2020 costs between 15,000-25,000. Gastric bypass is on the higher end, with the gastric sleeve and banding being on the lower end. I began to ask the following questions to start planning for the cost of my lifestyle change.

- Would I qualify for coverage with my insurance?
- How much out-of-pocket costs would I incur for surgery?
- How much would vitamins cost me monthly?

What would my monthly grocery bill be?

- How will this change affect my family?
- What are the after-effects of surgery?

Thankfully, my insurance covered the bulk of my surgery. The insurance process took several weeks to be verified and approved. For many applicants through insurance, it can take several months or sometimes even a resubmission. Resubmission requires a bariatric candidate to review and reapply for insurance if the requested items have not been appropriately submitted or more information is needed. Some insurance companies may require a candidate to maintain a log of meals for a specific amount of time; thankfully, I was not required to log my meals; however, I kept a log on the app My Fitness Pal as I started my bariatric journey. I was able to have the bulk of my surgery and clinical visits covered through my insurance company.

Regarding post-surgery costs, vitamins are not as costly as I had expected them to be. My price for vitamins is approximately $30 monthly. I shopped around several places, and you can find great discounts and deals online. I include protein shakes in my diet now, and they carry the bulk of my food cost. Many companies will send you a sample of their protein shakes to try before your surgery if you contact them via email or simply call and ask. Taking these proactive steps helped me to begin preparing for home care.

GUIDEPOST #7:

CARING FOR YOURSELF AT HOME

"Give me six hours to chop down a tree, and I will spend the first four sharpening the axe." - Abraham Lincoln

THE PROCESS (AFTER SURGERY)

Preparation is key to having a positive transition from the hospital to home. Taking the time to prepare is never time wasted, and you will feel a sense of relief and gladness that you did!

I prepped my home before surgery to have all the significant items that I needed. I stocked up on water, purchased hospital gowns, extra pillows for my bed at home, bandages, antibiotic ointment, MiraLAX, and other items (see checklist). I am a planner by nature, and I wanted to have things in place before returning home. I had picked up a starter amount of supplies so that I didn't need to go out unnecessarily the first week. My sister Nancy handled the majority of my home care. She was the best! I was advised not to lift over ten pounds for a few weeks in my home-care instructions, no driving while on pain medication, and no bending. I decided not to lift anything at all.

I was in "operation protect your pouch" mode, and so was Nancy. We agreed. We sat down and reviewed the home packet together, and I wrote down any questions that I had and any questions Nancy had to pose to my doctor. I cannot stress the importance of having a reliable support team. Nancy was my home caregiver while recovering. She helped me to stay disciplined and was incredibly kind throughout the process. If I dropped something on the floor during the day, Nancy assured me not to pick it up and that she would get it when she arrived. Nancy made sure that I did not have to worry about laundry, dishes, or cleaning. She was right there the entire time to make sure that I healed well. Having someone with your best interest in mind and a positive attitude makes a great deal of difference during the recovery process. Going through anything new and unknown can be extremely frustrating. Nancy's presence made home recovery calming and full of comfort, even when the days ahead were challenging.

I did not start vitamins right away. I started taking vitamins a week after out of sheer ignorance. Unfortunately, I could not locate instructions concerning vitamins in my home/release orders from the hospital or written anywhere. I am sure there was an assumption that patients knew to go ahead and start taking vitamins; however, this whole process was all new to me. I was afraid that I was going to make a mistake and wanted to handle everything correctly down to every detail. I ended up calling my doctor's office for clarity, and of course, they urged me to begin taking my multivitamins and calcium right away. I tried a couple of vitamins that just didn't sit well with my stomach and nauseated me. Most of my vitamins are taken in liquid or chewable forms. I learned with working with my regular care physician and other doctors to always request medications as liquids or chewable. Often, the doctors may by habit prescribe other rigid forms such as tablets or capsules that will not digest well for bariatric patients. Some professionals say that you can eventually just go back to taking solid tablets and normal medication forms. I disagree. Mentally, I do not want to go back to anything I was used to before surgery. Making modifications to medications is a reminder for me that I have had something done medically and internally. It also reminded me that I need to keep my life adjusted to be successful and thrive. Keeping my pouch healthy and protected was, and still is, my number one goal when I think about the medications that I take and the food that I consume.

I remember being very sore and uncomfortable coming out of the gastric bypass surgery. To my surprise, I was not in any unbearable pain. Keep in mind that everyone's pain tolerance level is different. Some who have undergone the same kind of procedure say that they felt as though they were hit by a truck when they came out of surgery! I am grateful that excessive pain was not the case for me. I was, unfortunately, on my menstrual cycle, which tended to be very discomforting. My doctors gave me adequate doses of pain medication that helped me tremendously with my pain. One of my supporters, Kathy, whom I mentioned earlier, advised me to stay ahead of the pain and not reject any pain medication whenever my nurse came in and offered it. I gladly accepted and followed that advice! I was given water, and two ounces of vanilla protein shake to sip each day during my hospital stay. The nurse did not rush me, but she asked me to get as much down as possible. I did not have an appetite, perhaps because I was very sore. I was in the hospital for three days. Before being released, I had to undergo a type of drink test to ensure no holes in my new stomach. My new stomach was then being referred to as my "new pouch." I attempted to drink as much as possible of the very offensive, white, thick matter before I was wheeled to the x-ray room. When I attempted to stand to have the x-ray taken, I was so dizzy that I had to be caught by the medical team before hitting the floor. Pressing past this moment was my first challenge.

I was very weak from surgery and only drank sips of protein shake and water in those three days. I was determined to steady myself and stand straight up while all the x-rays were taken. The experience was tough and painful. Later I received the results, and there were no holes to be found in my new pouch. My doctors did a phenomenal job conducting my surgery and keeping me informed about my progress during my time in the hospital. I was cleared to be released on day three. I went home with my medical packet that included my instructions for home care and next steps, my hugging pillow for my tummy, and a starter/sample of vanilla bariatric protein shake - all of which were provided by my doctors and medical team.

The bariatric shake that I was given in the hospital is what I continued drinking at home. For meals, I started sipping two ounces every two hours, along with an attempt at some water between. I will share more about my complications with water in the next chapter. Being back home,

I knew that I needed to remain active. I hit the pavement and started to exercise. Bariatric patients are encouraged to become active as soon as possible to prevent blood clots. I began walking less than .25 miles the first week home—which is just up and down the street on which I lived. Once I would get back to my home, I was exhausted!

Nevertheless, the short walk was my daily routine until I could build up my strength. Each day I would include more steps until I was able to increase the steps to a mile. Sleep comfort was also a part of my new regimen; therefore, I prepared my couch to be my bed since I had decided not to lie in a horizontal position for the first three months. I had heard stories of acid reflux for persons who were sleeping in a lowered, horizontal position; for this reason, I wanted to do as many preventative steps as possible to avoid any complications. My sister purchased a special pillow for me to sit up comfortably, and I camped out on my living room couch those three months. To my delight, I had very little reflux; thus, reflux ended up not being an issue for me. I was progressing well. I did not rush back to work after surgery. My doctor's office told me that I could go back to work after two weeks; however, my body had a slightly different schedule. I went back to work six weeks after my surgery date. I urge you to listen to your body and take as much time as needed to get back and adjust. I slept a great deal after the first four weeks of surgery (twelve hours a day). Apparently, I needed the rest because little things would take a lot out of me, especially walking. I had to train my body to get back into a routine. It took work! Even when you do not feel like moving, you have to push past the emotion and get active!

GUIDEPOST #8:

COMPLICATIONS AND HOW TO RESPOND

Nothing worthwhile is ever without complications. - Nora Roberts

Complications are par for the course whenever you have a weight loss surgery or a major procedure performed. Complications can be minor or severe, depending on how your body responds. Thankfully, I did not have severe complications after surgery. However, I experienced some of the more common challenges, such as taste and smell, constipation, light reflux, dumping, dry mouth, and depression.

The Senses

God gave all of us the wonderful gift of "the five senses": We can see, hear, touch, taste, and smell. Out of these senses, I was most challenged with the senses of taste and smell following surgery. The change in these two senses was new and different. My sense of taste and smell began to be more acute and heightened. My doctors and medical support team shared that my sense of taste and sense of smell could very well change. For instance, some of the foods, vitamins, and drinks that I liked prior to surgery, I was unable to eat or drink post-surgery. Many of the foods that I enjoyed had a taste and texture that my new pouch did not tolerate. For example, I loved my eggs scrambled hard, and somehow, no matter how little I attempted to eat, it would just come right back up! I eat hard-boiled eggs with no problems or challenges. The texture or how the egg was prepared was the difference. The chewable vitamins that I purchased prior to surgery I no longer could tolerate after surgery due to the strong smell and taste. The tolerance of certain foods and drinks were intolerable following surgery. My doctors warned me of the possibility of the change in my senses, and boy, were they right! My senses underwent a complete upgrade, and each sense had become extremely sensitive and heightened! I did not understand my doctor's warning beforehand.

At the beginning of this new phenomenon, I was in misery: My next challenge was with water. For the first three months, I could not stand to drink any water. The taste of any of the major brands of water made me gag and nauseous. I was able to drink protein shakes without complication. Not being able to drink water had me sincerely concerned since I knew that this challenge could lead to other difficulties in my body. I tried several brands of water, and I just could not hold any of them down. Each brand that I tried tasted like toilet water; neither could I stand the smell of those waters. Not being able to drink the primary source of nutrients to hydrate my body led to another complication — constipation, a condition which occurs when bowel movements become less frequent, and stools become difficult to pass. Constipation happens most often because of changes in diet or routine or because of inadequate intake of fiber. You should call your doctor if you have severe pain, blood in your stools, or constipation that lasts longer than three weeks (Cleveland Clinic). Whenever I felt as if I wanted to have a bowel movement (BM), "the movement" just would not happen because my bowels had hardened. My body would respond as if I needed to have a BM and emit the sensation of having to rush to get to the bathroom, only to find that I could not release anything. What a horrible feeling! Having become desperate for hydration and relief, I finally tried Fiji water, and this specific brand was no problem for me to drink and went down with ease. Also, I added Benefiber to green tea and sipped on it throughout the day. In addition to my desperate attempt to get rid of my constipation, I found a liquid Colace capsule, broke it open, and mixed it inside my Greek yogurt—BIG mistake! Colace is capsulated for a reason. And the reason is that it burns. At first taste, my mouth was lit on fire, and so was my throat!

The Colace burns when consumed outside the capsule and the taste is so extremely bitter that the mixture of the bitter taste and the sensation of burning immediately made me vomit. On a lighter note, I called my doctor's office, and the assistant shared with me that MiraLAX helped alleviate constipation; I added some of it to my water and Crystal Light. Taking the route of wisdom from my doctor, the professional advice helped to aid in relief tremendously! Along with constipation, I also had a slight encounter with acid reflux. Acid reflux is a common condition that features a burning pain known as heartburn in the lower chest area. This ailment happens when stomach acid flows back up into the food pipe. Also, for your information (FYI), Gastroesophageal reflux disease (GERD) is diagnosed when acid reflux occurs more than twice a week (HealthToday). To get ahead of the possibility of acid reflux symptoms, I chose to sleep sitting up on my couch for the first few months after surgery. None of the medical professionals shared that I take this measure. Still, I chose to camp out on my couch after hearing many patients in my support group who were bypass and sleeve patients mention having acid reflux badly, and especially, while lying down. I wanted to curb that part of my journey. Although I experienced only slight reflux symptoms, and my doctor prescribed medication to help with the symptoms, I still decided to sleep sitting up on my couch the first two to three months after surgery.

Dumping

Of course, the first few months were trial and error, and I called them "My Sick Patient" months. The process took several trial-and-error moments to determine how to identify the foods which my body could take in and digest without vomiting or having the feeling of nausea. I stuck mainly to protein shakes the first eight weeks after surgery. I attempted to go through the puréed stage—unsuccessfully—and ended up vomiting, no matter how fine I chopped up the veggies or beans in my newly purchased Ninja blender. I didn't force myself to go through the puréed stage. My body said, "No." Every time I introduced a new food, my body would reject it. I would spend more time in the bathroom vomiting than the time it took to prepare the meal! Once you go through a certain level of dumping, you lose the desire to eat, smell, or even think about food. Dumping syndrome after gastric bypass surgery develops when food gets "dumped" directly from your stomach pouch into your small intestine without being digested—two types of dumping syndrome that can take place: early and late. Early dumping happens ten to thirty minutes after a meal, and late dumping happens one to three hours after a person eats. Each has slightly different symptoms.

Early symptoms of dumping syndrome include nausea, vomiting, abdominal cramping, and diarrhea. These symptoms usually start ten to thirty minutes after you eat. Other early symptoms include: bloating or feeling uncomfortably full, flushing over the face, sweating, dizziness, or fast heart rate. Late symptoms appear one to three hours after you eat. They are caused by low blood sugar and can include: dizziness, weakness, sweating, hunger, fast heart rate, fatigue, confusion, or shaking (Health Line).

I happened to experience both stages of dumping for several months following gastric bypass. I slowly introduced small spoonfuls of Greek yogurt and Jell-O gelatin until my body could respond better to new foods. I thought I would not make it through this part of the journey because of how little I was eating and how much weight I was losing so rapidly. My medical support team at Southern Surgical suggested that I try Wendy's chili in month three. Having the chili was a life-saver for me. Before eating chili, I honestly thought that I had made the wrong decision about surgery because I was having such a trying time keeping food down, and I began to feel miserable. This was a challenging moment, and I wanted to end my mental misery! A friend reminded me that having this type of moment was normal and was only temporary and that "this too shall pass." If I could get past that particular moment, that pushing past it would be worth taking on in the long term. Even the best hikers find that the most challenging parts of their thru-hike journey are the exposure to severe weather conditions, unbalanced terrain, and high inclines. But determined hikers never give up. Just as the hiker (had to do), I had to continue on my path despite the changing conditions. I had the end of my journey in full view, and challenges are par for the course. At three months, I had lost sixty-seven pounds.

Dry Mouth

Dry mouth is also known as xerostomia. It occurs when salivary glands in your mouth don't produce enough saliva. This condition causes a parched or dry feeling in your mouth. It can also cause other symptoms such as bad breath, a dry throat, and cracked lips. Saliva is a necessary part of your digestion process. It helps moisten and break down food. It also works as a major defense mechanism to help your body maintain good dental health while protecting your mouth against gum disease and tooth decay (Health Line). As a bariatric patient, you may experience dryness in your mouth and nasal passages that may become very noticeable. Dry mouth is usually a temporary and treatable condition.

In most cases, you can prevent and relieve symptoms of dry mouth at home by doing one or more of the following: sipping water often, sucking on ice cubes, avoiding alcohol, caffeine, and tobacco, limiting your salt and sugar intake, and using a humidifier in your bedroom when you sleep. I used a humidifier and rinsed with *Bioteen* mouthwash my first couple of years following surgery for my relief of dry mouth. The *Bioteen* coupled with the humidifier, helped tremendously with dryness and kept my sinus pathways moist. Having the humidifier active during the day and at night allowed me to sleep and rest better and alleviated any restlessness due to dry air or the dryness I was experiencing in my sinus pathways.

Depression

I started to feel depressed during my third month, and depression recurred during month six. The changes that I began experiencing took more of a toll on me mentally. There were several that I just wasn't prepared to deal with emotionally. Thankfully, if you have a good doctor's office, you are connected with a psychologist that you are scheduled to see prior to having surgery and have scheduled sessions after surgery. During my third month, I remember feeling very low in my mental state after continuing to see all of the vitamins and medications on my kitchen counter each day. With what appeared to be little effect, I was popping vitamins all the time. I was also barely eating anything. As mentioned earlier, I skipped the puréed stage because I just could not hold anything down. Over time, I was able to eat a couple of spoonfuls of Greek yogurt or something similar, and I was done. Most aromas or scents nauseated me: perfumes, exhaust from cars, the minty taste of my toothpaste—you name it, I couldn't stand the smell, and I would get sick and vomit. After surgery, my sense of smell was keenly heightened, which I thought was the worst thing ever at the time (my keen sense of smell later turned me into a pretty great cook). I began to feel as though I were someone who was terminally ill. I seemed to "dump" so often the first three months that I lost all desire to eat. The process was so very frustrating and took a mental and physical toll on me.

Dumping, mentioned in an earlier guidepost, is the point at which you can experience vomiting and other symptoms when a food does not agree with you, or you eat too fast. At other times losing weight quickly, vomiting left me feeling physically drained. Seeing my body change so rapidly began to scare me instead of making me happy about the weight loss. I felt as if I was on a roller coaster. I wanted things to slow down, and it seemed like my weight loss was happening so fast and getting faster. I didn't like the feeling of being out of control. I thought I was gaining control of my weight, not losing control!

Wasn't that the reason why I had surgery? This didn't feel normal. After six months, I had reached my weight loss goal and was already down 125 pounds. But I was supposed to be happy, right? It doesn't always work that way. I tried to sabotage my weight loss as I continued to lose weight. I felt the need to control it, and I couldn't. All of these factors caused me to have depression. I was ready to stop, but my weight just kept dropping. It didn't help that people were asking me if I were sick and giving me their opinion (without knowing that I had had weight-loss surgery). People would say statements like: "Don't you think that's enough weight for you to lose? Darling, are you well? You don't want to lose any more weight. You should stop right where you are." Someone even told me how "bad I looked" and that I needed to gain weight instead of lose it. If some have pulled out a sandwich and handed it to me, I think I would have lost it at that point! Remember to keep in mind that it is your opinion of yourself that matters. People will always have or give their opinion. It is what you have in your head about you that counts.

Getting through the negative thoughts and feelings of depression took faith and positive self-talk. I had to quickly remind myself of why I was on this weight loss journey in the first place. I did not want to go down the path of other family members. I wanted to change the trajectory of my life. I leaned in hard on my faith and stayed fervent in prayer. I shared my feelings and thoughts first in prayer and asked God for guidance and wisdom. I openly shared my feelings with Him. I wrote down when I felt the feelings of depression and searched out why. In response to my soul searching, I made simple adjustments that helped significantly in my attitude about surgery. Since the medicines on the counter made me feel like a sick patient, I removed them and placed them in a cabinet instead of leaving them on the counter where I could see them each day. Also, I began sleeping in my bed again three months post-surgery. After my three-month hiatus, I enrolled in a nearby gym to include more exercise (outside of my typical walking routine) to be around more people and build momentum. I also started to be more active outdoors rather than engaging in indoor activities. The latter allowed me to smell the fresh air and sun on my skin and help push aside any negative feelings. I began to investigate more foods to eat that would be "pouch friendly" and visited http://theworldaccordingtoeggface.com. This website had numerous recipes to explore and to help me through my first few months!

One of the most significant contributors to better mental health was my daily affirmations and confessions. The affirmations helped to set the focus and pace for my days. I also contacted my clinical psychologist and shared where I was mentally. He gave me great insight into approaching my feelings and agreed that maintaining an active lifestyle and surrounding myself with positive, supportive people played a major role in good mental health. I also decided to create a "Do It Aimz" list. This list included the things I couldn't do at my highest weight that I now would be able to do at my new weight and size. Some of those things included: going to a park and swinging on a swing, buckling my seatbelt on an airplane without having to endure the embarrassment of asking for a seatbelt extender, joining the local softball team, riding a horse, taking a ride on a hot air balloon, and to hike a trail.

I have completed the majority of the activities on my list. I hope that when you are in a difficult spot or suffer the feeling of defeat that you steadfastly fight to gain your footing and push yourself out of the mental rut. Know when to call your support team when the struggle becomes unbearable to handle; I found that in some instances, and at my most trying times, it is just you and God on the journey – you're never alone. Combining all of these strategies proved to be the winning combination that pulled me out of depression and led me down a better path. I persevered, and you will too!

GUIDEPOST #9:

TAKING CARE OF YOUR BODY AFTER SURGERY

"The wall! Your success is on the other side. Can't jump over it or go around it. You know what to do." - Dwayne "The Rock" Johnson

Much work remains to be done after weight-loss surgery. A major part of the work is taking good care of your health and wellness. Since your physical body is the only one you have, you must take good care of it through exercise, physical activity, and mental wellness. Incorporating physical exercise is essential for long-term weight loss success. Furthermore, regular physical activity is one of the best things you can do for your body and overall health, specifically through physical exercise. Types of physical activity may include walking, swimming, running, biking, or working out at your local gym. I found that including physical activity each day immensely helped with consistency, discipline, and accountability—all of which are needed to accomplish your goals.

Carving out a specific time each day to exercise will coax you into a healthy course of action to follow. My daily routine began at 4:00 AM with a drive to the gym at 5:00 AM for a forty-five to sixty minute workout. However, I did not merely start working out after surgery. I began gym workouts before surgery so that I could start making the life changes needed to be successful at maintaining my weight loss. In the beginning, it was difficult. I felt every pound of my excessive eating and lack of activity. I felt the shame of my weight, and I had all of the fears of being a beginner. The difference this time was that I had more skin in the game, and I was more determined. I took the time to learn every machine at my local gym. If I didn't know how to use one of the machines, I would ask someone or the personnel to demonstrate how to use it properly. I became more familiar with my new environment and lifestyle. The more I practiced getting up in the morning and working out; the more natural and normal my new lifestyle became. Notice that I did not say that making the changes got any "easier." Even after dropping 145 pounds, I must confess that working out can be a challenge; however, it is a decision that I make each day.

We get to choose how successful or unsuccessful our journeys will be. Dr. Mehmet Oz (Dr. Oz) stated, "Be proactive. Carve out time in your schedule and take responsibility for being the healthiest person you can be. No one else is going to do it for you." I took time to get familiar with the gym prior to surgery because I wanted to prepare my body for all that it would undergo during and after surgery. My goal was to build endurance and put into practice a routine that I could keep. I wanted to feel the discomfort so that I could push past it and be familiar with what discomfort felt like. I didn't want the feeling of discomfort to be a huge shock for me when it was time to hit the ground running (literally!). Along my journey, I began to get more and more active by including swimming, dancing, gardening, weight lifting, and working out more vigorously. Having a solid workout routine and incorporating an active lifestyle is also great for mental health. A recent study done by the Harvard T.H. Chan School of Public Health found that running for fifteen minutes a day or walking for an hour reduces the risk of major depression by twenty-six percent.

In addition to relieving depression symptoms, research also shows that maintaining an exercise schedule can prevent you from relapsing. Exercise is a powerful depression fighter for several reasons. Most importantly, it promotes all kinds of changes in the brain, including neural growth, reduced inflammation, and new activity patterns that promote feelings of calm and well-being. It also releases endorphins, powerful chemicals in your brain that improve your mood. Finally, exercise can also serve as a distraction, allowing you to find some quiet time to break out of the cycle of negative thoughts that feed depression (Help Guide). Having a solid workout routine has several benefits, such as improving mental and physical health. Many people who get weight loss surgery may slack in routine workouts and experience heavy bouts of depression and excess skin.

SKIN

Loose skin is not something that you can necessarily avoid as a bariatric patient. Any rapid weight loss exceeding 100 pounds or more you can almost expect to result in excess skin. The good news is that you can be proactive and learn more about how your skin reacts to weight loss or weight gain, how to manage the loose skin, or to consider plastic surgery as a mile marker on your journey. The skin is the largest organ of your body, and it forms a protective barrier against the environment. The innermost layer of your skin consists of proteins, including collagen and elastin. Collagen, which makes up eighty percent of your skin's structure, provides firmness and strength. Elastin provides elasticity and helps your skin stay tight. During weight gain, the skin expands to make room for increased growth in the abdomen and other parts of the body. Pregnancy is one example of expansion. Skin expansion during pregnancy occurs over a few months' time, and the expanded skin typically retracts within several months of the baby's birth. By contrast, most overweight and obese people carry extra weight for years, often beginning as early as childhood or adolescence. When skin has been significantly stretched and remains that way for a long period, collagen and elastin fibers become damaged. As a result, they lose some of their ability to retract (Health Line).

Most bariatric patients usually gain most excess skin around the stomach and legs/thigh areas. I experienced the most loose skin on my legs, arms, and back. Those who have loose skin can experience challenges such as physical discomfort, skin irritation and breakdown, and an overall poor body image. What is more, excess skin can be uncomfortable and interfere with normal activity. A study of 360 adults found that this problem occurred most often in people who had lost 110 pounds (50 kg) or more (Health Line). After surgery, I experienced high discomfort in my underarm area and the inner thigh area of my legs whenever engaging in exercise. I began to chaff while attempting to run for short distances. I could not run over a mile before experiencing pain and irritation in those areas. I scheduled an appointment with my general care physician to get a consultation on how to combat the chaffing and for documentation purposes. My doctor suggested that Gold Bond powder be used to prevent chaffing and that I continue to use Vaseline to grease up before hitting the gym as measures to help with any discomfort. In a study of twenty-six women, seventy-six percent reported that their loose skin limited exercise mobility. What's more, forty-five percent said that they had stopped exercising altogether because their flapping skin caused people to stare (Healthline).

After my first encounter with chafing, I invested in a pair of black compression pants built for friction (much like football players wear). The compression pants kept the skin still and friction at a minimum. I also wore long sleeve compression workout tops that kept my body cool and lessened the irritation. However, I still had limitations. I could still run, but I had to stop after a mile, or I would experience chafing and sometimes even pain in my breasts from the constant movement. After three years of making do with creams and powders, I decided to have plastic surgery. One study found that of 124 people who requested plastic surgery to tighten skin after weight loss surgery, forty-four percent had reported skin pain, ulcers, or infections due to the loose skin. Loose skin from weight loss can also have negative effects on body image and mood (Health Line). I can certainly attest to the skin irritation and the negative effects it had on my body image.

On the surface, in these instances, everyone can seem to be normal and just fine in appearance. After losing the weight, I received a good many compliments on my figure and appearance.

No one knew, except my support team, that underneath my jeans were Spanx, and under long or ¾ length shirts were extra small camisoles to hold my skin in place so that I wouldn't chaff from daily activities. Underneath the camisoles were bras that I stuffed with socks in order to fill the cup. I usually get a lot of questions from ladies about the body and especially regarding breast changes with weight loss: "Will your cup size change?" The answer is, "Yes." I started my journey with a 42DD bra size. When I reached my weight loss goal of 145 pounds down, I was a 32B cup.

Needless to say, my breasts were as deflated as a latex balloon. The appearance of my breasts affected my view of myself and caused depression. My breasts, the body parts that made me feel most like a woman, were gone. The bra cup was only holding skin! I was probably actually an A-cup. It was extremely hard to look in the mirror each day and see all of the hanging skin from my breasts to my arms, legs, and back. It seemed as though that I had loose skin everywhere! Once I took off all the clothes and compression garments, I did not feel as if I were confident or beautiful. The skin looked horrible. I decided to make a change. I was going to have plastic surgery on my arms and breasts. Like the decision to have bariatric surgery, I went through the same research process to find an excellent surgeon to do the work. I followed a workout routine to prepare my arms and chest for surgery and to have some muscle definition. I wanted my heart to be in good shape as well and included a cardio plan. I followed a good solid plan for a year. In 2018, I had an arm lift and a breast lift with implants. Plastic surgery was on my list of items to "possibly do" if I couldn't deal with the skin. I placed in the plan from the beginning to revisit should I not be able to stand living with the excess skin. "Plan to go the distance" became my mantra.

HAIR CARE

We all love our hair and desire to take care of it to our best ability. With rapid weight loss, challenges with hair loss or hair texture can be an obstacle. Understanding your hair type, how to care for your hair, and determining preventive measures to take are important components to help to combat hair loss. Hair loss after bariatric surgery is very common and very stressful because we all want to achieve great weight-loss results and still have attractive hair. The hair loss associated with weight-loss surgery is called *telogen effluvium* and has to do with the normal hair growth cycle. The condition usually starts abruptly and very seldom lasts longer than six months. Human hair has a two-stage growth cycle. The growth phase is called *anagen*, and ninety percent of our hair follicles are in this phase at any given time. The resting phase is called *telogen*, which lasts about one to six months, with an average of three months. About five percent to fifteen percent of our hair is in the resting phase at any given time. It is also known that *telogen effluvium* has to do with stress to the body and hormonal changes that can occur. Due to the stress, more hair follicles can enter the resting phase. This is important because the hair in the resting phase at the time of surgery is most likely the hair you will shed.

The reason is that your hair sheds between one to six months after surgery (usually about three to four months). When the hair starts to grow again, the old hair follicle is released, and you lose hair. Sometimes the hair comes out before new hair grows (Dallas Medical). Prior to surgery, I spent much time researching and getting a good strategy and system to put in place to be successful. Hair was one of the things on my list of "How do I manage this?" One of the key parts of my strategy was that I stopped getting chemical treatments for my hair. Chemical treatments included coloring, relaxers, perms, etc. I stopped all treatments three months prior to surgery and began taking a multivitamin along with biotin. The amount to intake is based on your body weight/size.

My goal was to introduce my body to these new vitamins so that I did not go into vitamin overload post-surgery. I increased the amounts of biotin, D3, iron, and B12 after surgery due to the intake balance that occurs after having gastric bypass. During the time that I stopped all chemical treatments for my hair, I wore a sophisticated, customized, layered hair piece(s). Many hairstylists call this method "protective styling" for your hair. *Protective styling* is normally used when your hair has been severely damaged and needs time to rest and repair itself. I would also get protein hair treatments quarterly to keep my hair healthy while in its protective state. I waited three years after surgery before I began adding chemicals to my hair again. After that period of time, my professional stylist shared that my hair was strong enough to begin chemical treatments again. At the time of my bypass surgery, there was not any literature available to guide me through the hair care process. Believe me, I looked! I spent time in prayer and asked God for wisdom, insight, and a plan. My hair, after I took it out of the protective style, was fuller, healthier, and grew longer and thicker than it was before gastric bypass surgery.

GUIDEPOST# 10:

KNOW THYSELF

"Knowing thyself is the beginning of wisdom" - Socrates

One of the biggest challenges you will overcome in this bariatric journey is overcoming yourself. The challenge is the choice. The challenge is in the choices that you make each day: overcoming the temptation to hit the snooze button to get up for your workout or lie in bed for the next hour. The choice to have that slice of cake or decline it and opt for the small cup of coffee instead. If you loved food before surgery, you more than likely will have a love for food after surgery. You must adjust be successful. The same is true of exercise. If you are lazy about exercise before surgery, you could potentially carry that same behavior of being lackadaisical about exercise into your new lifestyle, unless you have a change of mindset. Jim Rhon, another one of my favorite thought leaders, said, "You have to change your mind to change yourself." I had to find the strength within myself to move forward with the choice I initially made to have surgery. That one choice turned out to lead to a series of choices that I would have the opportunity to make. I had a great support system in place, but they were not with me 24/7. I had to choose to make smart choices with or without the team present. I had to choose to get up at 4:00 AM to go to the gym to create space for my new lifestyle. Because I chose to get up at 4:00 AM, I also had to choose to go to bed early and on time. Practicing these behaviors is a cause and effect arrangement. One action impacts another. Rest is essentially important to healthy and consistent weight loss. I am not an after-work gym person. I'm better equipped in the morning to tackle a workout, as I have learned that about me. (You'll learn which practice works best for you too!) An early morning workout revs me up to start my day. After work or evening is strictly family time, and I have positioned my life to guard that time. The bright side is that you can win against the temptations and challenges that come along with change.

You must make positive mental shifts at each turn or change. This is the mental posture that you choose to take throughout your weight-loss journey. It's a mind that says: "I can do this." It's a mind that will embrace change and a new lifestyle. Your success will be at the level that you choose to make it.

This guide was created to help prepare you to maintain your long-term life change and shift your habits and behaviors to fit your new lifestyle. For successful and safe weight loss, this change will affect how you live your life—for the rest of your life. Everyone's journey is different and will have its own challenges. The decisions that you make as it relates to how you eat, live, exercise, and approach this new way of living life will determine your success. You have to make the decision to say, "This is it, this is what I'm going to do. And I'm sticking to it." I positioned my mind to say that I will not waste my meal opportunities on empty calories. Reaching the best levels of protein for my new lifestyle was and is essential, so I set goals daily. This behavior started BEFORE surgery. I had to build up a mindset and make decisions as to how I was going to live my life going forward. I COULD NOT remain the same. In my body or in my mind, things had to change. I cannot stress the importance of one who must "make up their mind" or the importance of forming decisions to make changes and to be committed and disciplined to those decisions.

As a bariatric coach, I have helped people rearrange their lifestyles and helped them to adjust when life introduced new challenges: family crises; job transitions; new baby; new move, new milestones, etc. Understanding that life will continue is important to embrace during your journey. Many will become discouraged and revert to eating comfort foods when life throws a challenge. I have been there. At one point of my journey, I was having back-to-back life obstacles: job loss, a health challenge, a sick mother placed in hospice and then our country being struck by Covid-19. In panic mode, I started trying to eat the pain away. Thankfully, I had disciplined myself enough throughout the years that my triggers kicked in. I not only had the triggers from surgery, but also had gained new habits, which I had practiced, that had now become my new normal. Our instinct is to go back to the familiar. My new familiar was a healthy lifestyle. The goal is to keep moving upward, no matter how tough the climb. No matter how arduous it gets, keep moving. I promise you that the panoramic view from the summit is worth the climb. Make it a great journey!

Success is not final; failure is not fatal: it is the courage to continue that counts. - Winston Churchill

MAKE IT A GREAT JOURNEY!

MILE MARKERS

Guide Post #1 Securing Your Why

Ask yourself the following questions to help find your path to why:

1. Why do I want to have weight loss surgery?
2. How successful have I been at my attempts at weight loss?
3. What is my current state of health?
4. Where do I see the state of my health in the next 5-10 years?
5. What are my healthy, natural, core eating habits?
6. Which surgery is the best fit for me?

Guidepost #2 Do Your Research

1. How much will surgery cost?
2. What is my Body Mass Index (BMI)?
3. What is the current state of my health?
4. Do I qualify for weight loss surgery?
5. Who's the best medical doctor in my area performing bariatric surgery?
6. Where do I want my surgery performed?
7. Where can I find good references for the doctor's offices?

Guidepost #3: Consult Others

1. Connect with professionals: a weight loss office/practice/surgeon
2. Ask successful others about their experience
3. Ask unsuccessful others about their experience
4. Watch YouTube videos with testimonials about weight loss surgery
5. Check out the testimonials on credible medical websites

Guidepost #4: Consulting Others

1. Who can I talk to one on one that has had weight loss surgery?
2. What are my current eating habits?
3. How do I currently view food?
4. What healthy changes can I make now?

Guidepost#5: Making the Decision

1. What thoughts are keeping me from making the final decision?
2. Is what I'm thinking or believing true?
3. What would make me more comfortable about making the decision?

Guidepost #6: Your Support Team

1. How would this new decision affect my family?
2. Who would be great supporters on my journey?
3. Would I qualify for coverage with my insurance?
4. How much out-of-pocket costs would I incur for surgery?
5. What would be the changes be to my monthly budget?

Guidepost #7: Caring For Yourself At Home

Home Preparation Check List

- Vaseline
- Gauze pads
- MiraLAX
- Benefiber
- Milk of Magnesia
- Extra Pillows
- Antibiotic Cream
- Water
- A small supply of vitamins (taste may change)
- A small supply of protein shake (taste may change)

Gastric Bypass Diet Plan Post Surgery

Phase 1: Protein Shakes

Duration: 2 weeks

Meal Plan: 2oz of protein shake per meal

Quantity: 6 meals per day (Example: 8AM, 10AM, 12PM, 5PM, 7PM)

Sip on water and unsweetened beverages between meals

Avoid carbonated beverages

Phase 2: Pureed

Duration: 2 weeks puréed

Meal Plan: 2-4 oz of pureed food with no chunks and soft to consistency, requires no chewing

Quantity: 6 meals per day

Phase 3: Soft Foods

Duration: Week 5-6 months

Meal Plan: Food to be tender, soft, and moist. No tough or dry foods

Quantity: 2-4 oz each meal, 3-4 meals per day, two snacks in between

Sip on water and unsweetened beverages between meals

Avoid carbonated beverages

Guidepost #8: Complications and How To Respond

"Do It _______________! (Your Name Goes Here)" Post Surgery Activity List

WARNING! When you get the opportunity to do these activities, you will be highly emotional if doing for the first time. But the sense of achieving and doing will help you to gain momentum to continue the journey

- Swing on a swing
- Take the stairs
- Do a pull-up
- Go shopping (new wardrobe required!)
- Join a local sports team or be a part of a sporting event
- Visit a theme park and ride all the weight limit rides!
- Take a flight w/out a seat belt extender
- Take a flight and sit in the middle seat
- Horseback Riding
- Kayaking
- Ziplining

- Parasailing
- Surfing lessons
- Paddleboarding
- Complete an obstacle course
- Hike a trail
- Run a marathon
- Sky Dive

Guidepost #9: Taking Care of Your Body After Surgery

Practice Good Habits

- Wait 30 minutes before and after eating, before drinking
- Take your time while eating. Allot 20 minutes to eat per meal
- Chew food completely and thoroughly (count chews if you must!)- do not swallow chunks of food
- After each bite, pause, and if necessary, put your fork down between bites
- Eat protein first at each meal, then vegetables, and if room, carbohydrates

- Steer clear of carbonated drinks: sodas, sparkling, or any beverage that has a fizz
- Eat when hungry - do not wait until you're at hell's end to eat
- Carry a protein snack or a protein shake with you at all times
- Practice keeping a bottle of water with you for sipping. This is your new attachment/accessory!
- Keep your medication in liquid, dissolvable, powder, chewable, patch, or soft gel forms
- Eliminate straw sipping or gum chewing
- Divide your daily calories into six small meals.
- Choose complex carbohydrates such as whole grains.
- Avoid foods high in simple carbohydrates, such as those made white flour or sugar.

DAILY GOALS

- 60-90 grams of protein
- 125-150 carbs per day
- Eight glasses of water/ liquids per day

- 45-minute workout

Note: Your goals here will change according to the demand or lack of demand that you place on your body and also your lifestyle habits.)

DAILY PRACTICES

- Take small bites of food
- Keep a high protein/low carb diet
- Take vitamins everyday
- Exercise to build muscle, so it burns fat!
- Don't drink while eating (wait 30 min before and after)
- Steer clear of carbonated beverages

BEGINNERS WORKOUT

- Walk 1 mile
- 1 Sit-up
- 1 Squat
- 1 Plank
- Repeat each day and add as you build endurance

Guidepost #10: Know Thyself

DAILY AFFIRMATIONS

- I am healthy; I am disciplined, I am whole
- I am fearfully and wonderfully made
- God perfects all that concerns me
- I am equal to anything and ready for anything
- I am self-sufficient in Christ's sufficiency.
- My best life is ahead of me
- I will not quit; I am determined to finish
- MAKE SMART CHOICES

GET BACK ON TRACK ASSESSMENT

- What foods do I have in my refrigerator or cabinet that I need to trash?
- Am I sticking to the correct portion sizes?
- Am I connecting with my accountability partners and being honest about my challenges?
- Am I exercising regularly?

GROCERY LISTS

GROCERY LIST 1: Week 1-8

Protein Shake

Jello

Chicken Broth

Minimal Mashed Potatoes (Puréed Stage and after/See Bariatric Meal Plan)

GROCERY LIST 2: Week 8 to 6 months

Premiere Protein Shakes

Jello

Light and Fit Greek Yogurt

Mashed Potatoes

Eggs

Chili

Water

GROCERY LIST 3: Gradually Added Items Over Time

Eggs

Tuna

Turkey Bacon

Salmon

Tilapia

Turkey (sliced and ground)

Rotisserie Chicken (Thighs)

Black beans

Lima Beans

Lentils

Cabbage

Collards

Frozen Mixed Vegetables

Grapefruit

Watermelon

Oranges

Apples

Strawberries

Blueberries

Greek Yogurt

Spinach

Brussel sprouts

Sweet potatoes

Cheese

Greek Yogurt

Premiere Protein Shake

Peanut Butter

Salsa

Tortilla Chips

Wheat Thins

Green Tea

Unsweetened Tea

FOODS TO AVOID

- Fried foods
- Fast Food
- Processed foods (i.e.hot dogs)
- High fructose/sugar content
- Carbonated beverages

CPSIA information can be obtained
at www.ICGtesting.com
Printed in the USA
FSHW021909140221

9 780578 819280